My Punished Mind

My Punished Mind

◆

A memoir of psychosis

David C. Boyles

iUniverse, Inc.
New York Lincoln Shanghai

My Punished Mind
A memoir of psychosis

iUniverse, Inc.

For information address:
iUniverse, Inc.
2021 Pine Lake Road, Suite 100
Lincoln, NE 68512
www.iuniverse.com

ISBN: 0-595-30494-X

Printed in the United States of America

This book is dedicated to those who have had similar experiences as I. To those who are not able to put into words their horrible experiences; so that others can possibly understand what it truly means to be psychotic.

Thank you Michael, my brother, for being there for me more than anyone else was, during this horrid, life-shattering time in my life.

Contents

PREFACE—copy of medical/hospital record

Admission: 3/30/2001
Discharge: 4/10/2001

This 31-year old single white male is admitted for the first time to the psychiatric unit under Section 9.39 of the Mental Hygiene Law, the circumstances described as "Danger to self".

This is a 31-year old male who apparently was having some extreme religious thoughts, which were pre-occupying him to a point where he was unable to cope with them.

The patient reported not feeling good, having stomach cramps, and felt he had done something terrible. The patient was brought to the Emergency room by his step-father, up to Emergency room parking lot and then resisted coming in. The police were called to bring him in under section 9.41 and their statement indicates—"Boyles was in the E.R. parking lot with his step-father. Boyles came to the hospital on a voluntary basis. When he reached the parking lot at the E.R., he refused to come in. Boyles was acting irrationally and refused to talk with officers. Boyles was screaming he needed to go be saved. He states Boyles has been acting suspicious."

According to the family, the patient left Florida a few days ago, he stopped to visit in VA Beach and called to tell them he had done something terrible. He questioned Jesus Christ and now "He is punishing me". He can't eat, can't sleep. His brother got on the phone to tell them that he has not been sleeping, eating, and that the patient was on the way to visit his family in NY.

The following evening he showed up at his Mother and step-father's place and told them, "I am a born again Christian". He began crying and moaning since arriving. They observed him talking to himself and reading the Bible, according to his step-father. He reported, "David has never been very religious" that he knows of.

A couple of years ago, the patient is reported to have thought he would be abducted by UFOs, and that the world was coming to an end. And for the past few weeks he has been dwelling on his Father who passed away 23 years ago. The night of admission, after dinner, he asked his step-father to bring him to the hospital, stating—"I need to go get help". And on the drive to the hospital he was praying and not making any sense at all. Making religious statements then as they drove closer he began screaming in the car. He began fighting with his step-father who went to get security. On seeing security he became calm. And when sister and brother came in, he became combative again. The police were called for him to be escorted to the Emergency room and Crisis Center. The patient tried to run from the door, security had to restrain with the ER staff and medicate him with Haldol 5mg. and Ativan 4mg. He then began crying, wanting his Mommy. His step-father asked for the patient to be admitted and reported that he has known him since he was little and he has always analyzed things but "I have never seen him like this". They were concerned what could happen if they took him home. He told his Mother that he had a vision of his dead Father and he was going to show her what he looked like. Mother didn't know what he meant.

Treatment plan: Continued involuntary hospitalization, placed on Haldol 5mg. a.m and H.S. and Depakote 250 mg. twice per day.

Admission Evaluation:

The patient is calm and he states he is feeling good and he would like to be discharged and initially he is reluctant to discuss any mental problem and tells me that he never had any treatment and does not believe he has a mental problem. When further inquired—about his thinking, he slowly opened up and reports that he tends to be an obsessive person and two months ago he started to write a book and over and over he was concentrating on it and then suddenly thoughts popped out on him. He reports to have had religious thoughts, and says he has started reading the Bible and also heard voices of good and evil. He reports while he was driving up here from VA Beach there was a constant battle between the good in the front of the head and the evil in the back and going back and forth, "crawling like a worm". He also reports that for weeks he has had a lot of thoughts going through his mind and has been recalling all his past, which he has been trying to write. He also has been preoccupied with his Father who is deceased for 23 years and had not been close. He reports that he has not been eating or sleeping because of his pre-occupation with God and thoughts on his mind.

The patient reported that he had been laid off from work two months ago as an aircraft electrician but denied it had anything to do with his illness.

The patient reluctantly agreed that he has a problem that needs to be treated and agreed to take medication. Even though he voiced desire to be discharged, he was generally cooperative and after initial resistance did not present a problem. Arrangements were made to meet with his Mother and problems discussed in terms of need for continued treatment once better, upon discharge.

The patient denies any abuse of alcohol or drugs and also denies family history of mental illness.

The patient was placed on Risperdal with Depakote with good results and remission of racing thoughts, improvement in sleep as well as appetite. His grandiose thoughts also subsided. The patient had some tremulousness and muscle rigidity due to Risperdal, but treated with Cogentin; with improvement in sleep, appetite, and remission of manic and psychotic symptoms. With the patient's continued cooperation, it was felt that he could be converted to a voluntary status, which he accepted, and used privileges well, leading to a therapeutic visit which was successful.

The patient understood the need for continued psychiatric treatment and that he will stay on medications.

Mental status examination:

Patient is found to be alert, calm, cooperative with no agitation and reports hearing voices as well as belief of God having influence on him and unable to stop his thoughts.

He does not present any pressure of speech or flight of ideas and describes himself to be an obsessive person who likes to analyze things. He is oriented in all three spheres and affect is appropriate.

Diagnosis according to DSM-IV: Schizo-affective disorder.

Discharge Medications: Depakote 500mg., Risperdal 2mg., Cogentin 1mg.; twice per day.

INTRODUCTION

The first time that hospital report was read to me, I was sitting in the nurse's office in VA Beach. It was a month or so after I had been stabilized from my first relapse. I had a hard time comprehending it as I nodded in agreement that is was 99% accurate.

A year and a half later I went back to the hospital and signed for my rights to my own personal copy. When I finally had it in my hands, I still couldn't read it thoroughly (without anxiety and "thought blocking").

There is a lot of stigma and misunderstanding about mental illness in our society. There have been many times that I have wanted to openly talk about my problem to others to give them an insight to something they may never have heard about or understood correctly. There are not enough books published that are first hand accounts of psychosis. I have written this book to clarify the reality of what it means to have a mental condition and what the symptoms were and are like, first hand.

The diagnosis Bi-polar and Schizophrenia came into my life in April of 2001, at the age of 31.

When I asked the Doctors *why?*—they couldn't give me an explanation that made any sense to me (at the time). I was told—why does someone develop diabetes or cancer?

These unfortunate illnesses just happen, *without a reason.*

This is my memoir of a sequence of events during a time frame of over several weeks being in a state of euphoria. But then my elation turned into persecution from God for having questioned the Bible. I went from being in heaven one week, to thinking that I was dying the next. My mind took me on a journey that is explained by science, but is (sometimes) still questioned by religion. It took away over a year from my life, until I was medicinally stabilized and then able to finally accept the condition and move on with my life. **I never expected this horrible, life-altering experience.**

ONSET OF EUPHORIA IN FLORIDA

Before the "breakdown" I could have been very easily described as an idiosyncratic person. I was very eccentric to most people who knew me and met me. I was a heavy drinker in my 20s (and now I know why—I was self-medicating). I was heavily into the UFO phenomenon. I had been pretty much ever since high school. Lifting weights (working out) had been a main hobby of mine too. I was always very shy and had a hard time associating with others. But then something happened.........

There wasn't an exact point in time that it happened, but it did. Sometime just after the New Year, in 2001, was the onset of the condition. I was living in St. Augustine, Florida and was in a relationship with my girlfriend of over two years.

I began reading self-help books, reminiscing about my very early childhood.

Memories of fear and confusion were mostly on my mind. With my girlfriend at the time, we were talking a lot about the things that were on my mind concerning my relationship with my real father who died when I was eight. I kept reading self-help books. I wasn't satisfied completely. Was there more to read? I started to be *obsessive, over-analytical, and extreme* about the reading that I was doing. My views and feelings about living changed for the better. I was having what I labeled a *spiritual awakening* for how good it felt to "understand" a little more about what I never thought through thoroughly (about the first eight years of my life).

When my emotions started to amplify, I immediately labeled myself as being "blessed". I turned to religion/faith for answers. But I wasn't getting the answers I was expecting. Watching church shows became an obsession. My mind was full of so many thoughts and views of what life is really about, that I began to write a book. I began writing about my views on the societal systems around me. But it emphasized mostly on religion. It was a different kind of book, meaning the exact opposite of the way things were (in my view). I was bashing religion/faith for not telling me what I was experiencing; because the religious leaders on the TV were telling me to put everything into God's hands, to not figure things out for myself. I had a hard time accepting that. I was experiencing so many emotions on my own from all the reading I was obsessively doing. And for over a week or more, I continuously watched church channels and was writing my book at the same.

Before I got my expected lay off from my job I was already slipping into the euphoria of the condition. I was telling those close to me how great I was feeling. My girlfriend at the time was obviously the first. She loved it of course seeing me in such a great mood. I then labeled it as "my heart opened up". I felt pressured to keep talking about how good I was feeling. My thoughts were very dominating. When I went to visit with my Grandma, I couldn't keep to myself about how good I was feeling. I would talk about my book that I was writing. I spoke of all the ideas in my head. I dominated most of the conversations. She complimented me for talking the way I did. I had so many things to say. *I was so "deep" philosophically and spiritually.*

I wanted to read the Bible to try and understand what I had never read before. I was feeling so good that I wanted to know God. When my girlfriend and I read the first few pages of the Bible together, we questioned just about everything we read. We got confused and actually disturbed. A day or two later I remembered the questions that aroused in me from reading the Bible that I decided to read it by myself. I was confused at: the order of creation of man and then woman; the forbidden tree of knowledge (of good and evil); the shame and covering of nakedness, and then being punished; and God having no regard for Cain's offering.

Then the flood was inflicted, and soon after, the tower of Babel incident. God was mad and kept taking away from humanity. The more I read the more confused I got. My whole concept of what I had always believed about God started to change. I never made it past the first several pages. I started to over analyze the concept of "inside out" from the word seed being used in the scriptures. I kept breaking things down and questioning. The continuous covering of nakedness was puzzling me. While I kept trying to make sense of my bewilderment from reading, a profound revelation came to me while reading over again the Adam and Eve incident of eating the forbidden fruit. When I re-read the words "and they saw themselves", the interpreting meaning that came to my mind was—know thyself. Right when that came to mind I went into a "trance": my heart started pounding fast and hard, I began weeping excessively and loudly, and my thoughts raced religiously (literally). *I had a feeling that was from beyond my control.* The episode lasted about a minute. And from that moment on, I believed I had "found" God.

Now I had been "touched by God"; and already being euphoric, it was wonderful. I went down to the beach one afternoon and just stood there on the rocks and observed "life". I was "one with life". Everything made sense. I became so elated that I almost started to cry. And right in front of the others nearby. I wanted to scream out loud—"Isn't life beautiful?"

I began calling my brother in VA Beach constantly. I wasn't able to hold a conversation without crying, from being so emotional. I told him that I had found God and that he "touched me" while reading the Bible. I emphasized a message that I received from God. It was to "Live". But it's the way I said it to him, which he still reminds me to this day about.

I also called a friend to tell her to read the same verses from the Bible about Adam and Eve eating the forbidden fruit. I *insisted* that she do it, because something would happen to her if she did. It happened to me. {About a year later she told me she had read it over and over and nothing happened. She told me that she suspected from that conversation that something was "different" about me—no shit}

I was obsessively watching church channels and writing my book at the same time. I would constantly call my girlfriend at her job and tell her how good I was feeling. Eventually she got tired of me making such big deals out of normal things (to her and everyone else).

For a couple of nights I would go to sleep with a "conversation going on (in my head)". I would be talking to my deceased father in the "spirit world". I would also be analyzing good and evil.

I woke up one morning and the first thing that was "said to me in thought" was that 'you are one with God'. An overwhelming sensation of euphoria came over me and I began crying. It was too much. I couldn't handle it. By the second or third morning, it was "indescribable". I just lied in bed, still, and cried, as the elation took over my body. My thoughts were dominating everything. It was like a constant conversation. When I made it out of bed and into the bathroom, I was standing in front of the sink and mirror. Tears were running down my cheeks from crying, my nose was running, my forehead was flushing, and I was also drooling. I was terrified at the feeling that was overtaking me. I was staring at myself in the mirror asking, "what is happening to me?" My thoughts were non-stop. The concept of "inside out" was profound. I looked over to the bed and started to analyze where I was. I realized I had not been dreaming anymore. When I was sleeping, I was at peace. When I was awake, I existed. The water was running through my fingers and glistening brightly. My awareness was at full alert. I dropped to my knees and screamed at the top of my lungs, "I exist, I am in heaven." I kept screaming with absolute elation and joy flowing through my body. I was in Nirvana. My mind raced with thoughts I can't even describe. When the episode was over, my senses were enhanced. God had made my senses more perceptive for this existence.

I walked outside to leave and talked to my neighbor on the way out, telling her that I had just had an experience with God. I stopped to admire a flower on a tree, by smelling it and touching it. "Everything" seemed richer to my perception. When I got to my truck, and before getting in, I remember looking up at the sun and thinking to myself, "why is the sun gold/yellow and the cover of the Bible black?" Soon after, I got the idea that I was going to have to build a shrine for my morning wake-ups, so that I could scream with rejoice in private.

Another time, I remember looking at the Bible on the table and watching the preacher on the TV and thinking how the Bible was a gateway out of this world; to keep you/me away from enjoying this life.

I was compelled to speak to any preacher I could find at any church. I had so many questions (from questioning the Bible). I needed some answers. I was on a mission. I went into a Cathedral in downtown St.Augustine. There wasn't any preacher/priest available to talk to at the time. So I walked around a bit analyzing my observations according to my thoughts. The extravagance of the interior of the cathedral was impressive. I remember thinking how it was all just an illusion of someplace that doesn't exist. I was in heaven and this was just an attempt to keep you and me from enjoying this life.

Another day came, and it was a beautiful morning to wake up to. I was heading down to the beach, but was suddenly distracted to the lighthouse as I was driving by. So I decided to turn in that direction and go visit it. I am afraid of heights, so it took some time going up the stairs. When I reached the top I was afraid and amazed at the same time. My thoughts were analyzing everything. I perceived my view as "being in heaven". Everything was in an expression of inward to outward. As I stood there, at one point I got the feeling as if my soul had found its place and jumped out of me. It startled me so, that I literally dropped down to sit down to catch myself. And when I would lookdown, the ground rushed up at me. I acted like a little boy the whole time I was up there. I even got the "watch lady" to walk me around the circumference, so I could leave having accomplished something while I was up there.

I was on a mission of "self discovery and life revelations", so I wanted to share it with everyone else. Now that I had been unemployed for a while, I had extra time to go back to NY and visit with my family. But first, I was going to go to VA Beach and visit with my brother, on the way to NY.

GOING TO VISIT MY BROTHER IN VA BEACH, WITH PSYCHOSIS SETTING IN

I was feeling physically terrible the morning I left for VA Beach, to go visit with my brother. I hadn't vented my "morning wake up in heaven". As I was driving, I would start to cry for no particular reason. My thoughts had taken over. I was starting to get the impression that I had to keep mumbling and make noise verbally to feel better; and I did for a little bit. I was analyzing "inside out" continuously. Then the songs on the radio started to be singing directly to me. There was a messaging theme from all the songs. I was supposed to choose. I was stuck in between two worlds. The song "Again" by Lenny Kravitz, was God singing to me. Another song that I remember very well, having 'special meaning from God', was, "Follow me" by Uncle Kracker. Things in the environment were taking on new meanings. I noticed black birds flying in circles in the sky. It was a symbolism to me, of evil waiting to catch its prey.

Now I was considering myself to be a born-again Christian and was going to start wearing a cross (medallion) in honor of what I was experiencing from God. All of my thoughts were religious in nature and non-stop. I would tune into religion-preaching channels and listen continuously. *It was a very emotional drive.*

When I got to my brother's apartment there was an "emotional block". When I went to hug my brother an impression came over me saying I wasn't allowed to feel love anymore. I felt very uncomfortable. My brother sensed something was wrong with me. But I answered him that I was fine, when I wasn't. When we went to the Tavern to visit his girlfriend, I was an emotional mess. I couldn't stop crying.

In the morning we went to breakfast. I was hungry, yet my stomach ached with pain for not wanting food. I was only able to eat half of my meal. Later that day we went out for dinner. I was so confused with my appetite. Hungry, knowing I needed to eat, yet I couldn't. I was only able to eat just a few bites. The food didn't sit in me comfortably. *I was aching all over.* I realized that I had to start apologizing (to God). I was *not* supposed to have done all that questioning of the Bible (in Florida). My elation had turned into **extreme** *guilt and punishment.* I told my brother that I had to do "something" when we got back to his apartment. When we were there, I turned on the radio and turned up the volume, to drown out what I was going to do. I dropped to my knees and started screaming, "I'm so sorry" (to God), for forgiveness. My brother looked at me in fear; I didn't care, I had to do it. He went back into his room and left me alone.

Over the next couple of days I was only able to eat a few bites of food at a time, because I would get sick from eating. I went to a fast food restaurant one morning to get a breakfast sandwich. While I was there it seemed as if everyone was giving me strange looks. People's faces were turning a little disturbingly disfigured. When I drove back I noticed a man walking with a strange, crooked walk. I never had seen anyone walk like that before. The more I looked, the worse it got.

There was a night that I lied down to sleep, but I couldn't. My mind was racing with thoughts. And the sad part was that it was getting full of deep *dark* thoughts. Some of the thoughts that I can remember were: I was going to become a vampire; never see the sun again; never see my family again; never be involved sexually with women again. My thoughts were in fast forward. And they seemed as if they were erasing away. I became so inundated with fear at this point that I got up from the couch and crawled into bed with my brother. I started talking to him. Telling him how sorry I was (for whatever reasons—I don't remember). Then the phone started ringing very late at night. It was "evil" calling, to come and get me. I was supposed to answer it, to accept my fate. I obviously couldn't do it. {Would you have?}[My brother said it was one of his girlfriend's friends calling. I wasn't able to be convinced of that]. I think I dozed off for a couple of hours, but was woken up to thoughts again of having to apologize to God.

It was very early in the morning, just after sunrise. I got up, threw on my clothes and coat, and walked down to the beach. I staggered to the edge of the water and dropped to my knees. I looked around to see that I was alone, and then started begging for mercy from God. I became frantic and was yelling up at the sky. The harder I screamed, a *little bit* of relief came. A couple and their dog were coming, so I stopped, until they passed. I begged some more. I felt a *little bit* of physical relief, so I then stopped. I walked back to the apartment and lied back down on the couch to try and sleep.

I decided one afternoon to go to a church and talk to a preacher/pastor/reverend, whomever was first available. When I went into the back office to talk to the pastor, my mind was full of questions, but I didn't know where to begin. I don't remember the conversation too well, but I know I was extremely emotional and started to cry. I had been "touched by God" and didn't know how to explain it.

I told him that God had shown me a glimpse of heaven. He then told me, "so, what do you want, where do you want to go (when I die)? He led me in a little prayer, and I was crying the whole time. While my eyes were closed I could see a silhouette of a person. I was thinking, was it Jesus? When I calmed down, we left the room and he gave me a mini-tour of the church and invited me back to future services. He also gave me some literature to read. I left and went back to the apartment. I was non-stop talking to my brother about my visit at the church. He didn't know what to think. I was never a religious, church going person.

While I was reading from the Bible one afternoon, I started hearing noises. There was a squeaky spot in the floor of his mini-kitchen, when anyone stood there. It started to make that noise when no one was there. A spirit/Jesus was there, making the floor squeak. I started to ask him for relief of my pain. All of my thoughts were religious.

I was lying around in misery. I felt physical pain throughout my body.

Later that day as I lied there on his couch, I got the overwhelming sensation that I was dying. So as a way to accept it, I had to call home and say goodbye to my Mom and step-dad. My Mom wasn't there at the time, so I talked to my step-dad. From what I can remember, I told him that I was being punished by God for having questioned the Bible. I remember he said, "What?—People have been questioning the Bible since it was first written." I told him that I wasn't able to eat or sleep right. I was crying the whole time out of fear. He told me that I should go to the hospital for help. So when my brother came back he took me to the hospital. I checked myself in. I felt a little safer. I was taken into a room and questioned by a lady with a clipboard. I told her that I had been reading self-help books and my mind was full of thoughts. I was very emotional. She said she could read my face, and tell something was wrong. I was hungry so they brought me a sandwich and soda. I was able to actually eat something. When she left the room for a little while, I lied there and I was thinking again. I started to think about my real father and started to cry. My brother came over and consoled me by patting my back. I stopped after a few minutes. Then I started thinking about my brother being there and I hadn't seen him in a while and started crying again. I lied there in the fetal position crying like a little boy. *I was very emotional.* I eventually stopped crying. A second lady with a clipboard came in and tried to talk to me. The first thing I noticed about her was that she was wearing a cross on her necklace. She wasn't treating me the same as the first lady. She didn't seem as compassionate. {I look back on that moment, and if I had something about her wearing the cross, they might have realized that I was analyzing things "differently".} My brother was a little upset. He said that the second lady wanted to send me off to the state hospital and pump me full of drugs. Well eventually the first lady came back in to talk to me briefly and give me a couple of pills, called Zanax. I was told to take them, to help me sleep. When my brother and I were leaving and walking through the parking lot, I was emphasizing how much better I felt. We stopped off at the restaurant and I was telling everyone that I had a nervous breakdown. Unfortunately, I was actually chuckling about it. When we got home it was late and time to go to bed. I didn't take the pill. I figured I didn't need it, since I felt a little better.

When morning came, I woke up to feeling bad again. The one lady Doctor gave me a number to call her the next day if I had any problems. I was, so I decided to call. A young girl answered who kept telling me that the lady I was calling was unavailable. I remember very well that I was having intrusive thoughts at that point telling me "people don't help you, only God can". I wasn't able to focus my perception.

My Mother called and asked what the heck was going on with me from being at the hospital the night before. I just remember telling her that I had a nervous breakdown and laughing it off.

It was my last night there. I was leaving for NY in the morning. My brother let me sleep in his bed, while he slept on the couch. My mind was full of thoughts. It was non-stop thinking. I lied there in a state of physical euphoria. I can describe it as "lying on a bed of clouds". I was thinking about all the new good things that were going to be happening in my life. I was going to start going to church and lead a (new) good life. And a(n) (irrational) thought came to me, to support my new thinking—I was not going to touch myself and ever masturbate again. My new sex-life was going to happen after I got married; so abstinence [even to myself] was the only solution. But suddenly I was thinking too much and I was *not* supposed to be thinking these thoughts. I then saw a "pattern/face with different colors" forming above the bed. It was turning red, mad and horrific. God was mad at me for all that thinking. I was getting "the message" that I had to get up and go into the next room and get the Bible and bring it back into the bedroom and start reading again, to "understand" it. So I did. I closed the door and then sat in the middle of the bed. I didn't pick a particular page. I just opened it and started reading. I *had* to focus and concentrate. I was getting physical sensations of elation inside my head, running from the top down. God was touching me with his love. I was crying the whole time. Mucus was running from my nose and dripping on the pages. Fear and joy dominated me. I *had* to do this until it was enough (which just happened when I stopped). When I lied back down to try and sleep, I saw "white figure/formations" and then "colorful patterns" appearing and then disappearing. No two were alike. God was showing me glimpses of heaven. I was calmed down at this point and I finally fell asleep. But it was only for a few hours, and definitely not comfortably.

GOING TO NY TO VISIT MY FAMILY, BEING PSYCHOTIC

When I had left my brother's apartment that morning for NY, I had a lasting thought that I was going home to die. I felt in despair.

Religion was occupying my mind constantly. Somewhere along the drive I suddenly got a direct link to God and Jesus. I felt a physical sensation in my brain. I could feel my brain "working". A "signal" could be felt moving all around inside my head. I could feel the signal moving back and forth, from the front to the back and vise versa. Yes and Good answers were in the front of my head and No and Bad answers were in the back of my head. I began asking questions and was getting answers. Unfortunately, I don't remember the questions [sorry]. But as I was lovingly conversing with God, "another me" was budding in and making rude and bad comments. I didn't like what was being said so I would bite my tongue every time a bad comment was made. The thoughts that were going through my head were amazing. Some of them were: I was going to perform miracles for God; I was going to become a preacher; I was going to sing in the church choir......everything was religious based in thought.

I suddenly got a significant revelation that I was now turning into a man. My voice was to change deeper. So I started screaming at the top of my lungs. I was screaming so hard, that I tasted blood in my throat. When I realized I was still driving, "something said" to maintain control.

It was slowly becoming darker because the sun had set. When I looked off to my left I noticed a dark cloud formation in the sky. It appeared to be emerging from the "aspect of the approaching night". It was evil/demonic as it was forming. The more I stared at it the more it developed. I was now seeing things in nature from the "spirit world". And a "message" I got was—and you will know/see good and evil. I was then getting the physical sensations in my head again. My forehead was "beaming" at it, while the back of my head was tingling. A dominating thought was that I was going to be facing a war when I got to NY.

As I continued driving, the headlights of the cars from the opposing direction were shining excessively bright and being interpreted as another "contact from God".

I was just a few miles from the house when I got the "transaction" from God. I was to transfer energy from me to my Mom through a hug, to prove God's existence. In return I was to see a vision of my deceased Father in heaven. To me this was a revelation that 'God works in mysterious ways'. So I started to store the energy up in my chest that God was feeding me. The closer I got to the house the stronger it became. I was screaming for more, I was hysterical. (Remember that I was driving at the same time.) When I arrived, I jumped out of my truck and went storming into the house. My little brother was in the back living room watching TV. I asked where the parents were. He said they were out for dinner. I approached him and went to hug him. When I did so I asked him if he felt "the energy", he said, "no". I realized it had to be with my Mother, as originally planned. I started walking around the house in a frenzy—"I was talking to my thoughts". I remember how "invincible" I felt physically. I went into the bathroom and looked at my eyes to see how red they were. But they weren't red. Having not slept a normal nights sleep in about a week was the only problem that I could rationalize at the moment.

I was anxious to see my Mother and do "that thing" for her and I. Suddenly they were home. I ran outside to meet them. I was breathing heavily. I was at the top of the stairs looking at them, all worked up. I remember they just stopped and look at me in wonder (of course). I had to calm down. I wasn't supposed to scare them. When we walked back in the house I started talking to them about my views on life, and how I was now a born again Christian. My step-dad replied back saying something like—we won't have you pushing your (new) beliefs on us. While I was standing in the kitchen, I could see "things/figures" looking in the front windows. I was getting the impression they were trying to get in, to come and get me. But I ignored them. I was hungry, so I heated up some food and sat down to eat. But I had to pray first. I blessed the food and it went down tastefully. I could hear my Mom in the corner of the room saying to my step-dad into the next room a few things, one of them was, "he is talking to himself and crying". After I ate I had to do stuff. *I couldn't sit still.* I went and got the Bible and started reading from it. I was then compelled to bless the house. I started in my Mom's room. As I stood in my Mom's room reading from the Bible, I could hear her asking me, "who was I?". That I wasn't acting like her son. I was too focused. I paid no attention. I had to bless the entire house, room by room. While I was upstairs in my little brother's room reading, the floor started to shake lightly and there was a light rumbling noise. "Hell" was shaking beneath the house because I was there 'blessing the house'. {The shaking and rumbling was from the downstairs TV. My little brother had turned it into surround sound}. Then I started hearing noises in the bathroom and the other rooms. The "spirits" were making their presence known. I had to silence them. I had the power to do so. My forehead felt like it was glowing. So I used it to silence the noises by sticking my head in the dark rooms while I shouted at the noises to be quiet, in the name of Jesus. After doing this, I went back down stairs. While I walked down the stairs I could feel my head tingling in the back, the "evil" was behind me. Then my parents told me to try and get a good nights rest. My little brother wasn't around anymore {I guess I scared him away, obviously}.

I eventually calmed down and tried to watch TV. But while I was watching the weather channel, "the snake"(from the Bible) formed itself in the clouds. It was coming to get me.

When I went to bed, I went to bed in **absolute fear**. I was upstairs all alone. The "evil" was coming to get me again. When I went to lie down, something touched my foot. I completely wrapped my body and head with the blanket to protect myself from the "spirits of the night". EVERYTHING was out to get me. I heard every little noise in the house. I noticed every shadow. *I lied there in complete fear*. I started to mumble to myself (all night) saying, "I'm so sorry (to God)". Then I could feel my brain twisting and turning. God was doing "something" to my mind. I just lied there helpless as it happened. I do not remember sleeping that night. The next thing I knew the sun was coming up.

During the day I was restless. I remember going downstairs and trying to talk to my Mother; but I don't remember a damn thing I said to her. I realized I had to try and get some sleep, since I didn't sleep worth a damn the night before. So I went back upstairs to lie down. I think I dozed off for maybe an hour or two, but was woken up to a screeching noise and the feeling as if something jumped into me. The only thing that made sense to explain what had just happened at that moment was to think back at that day at the lighthouse. I remembered the feeling of my soul jumping out of me, so now something "bad" had jumped into me. How horrible!!!

Thoughts of fixing what I had done wrong now took over. A solution came to mind. Now I had to re-read the Bible to "correct it". I had marked it all up with notes and questions from prior reading and questioning (in Florida). First, I *had* to erase *all* the marks I wrote throughout the whole book. I **crucially** made sure of it. Then I *had* to re-read all the sentences/phrases *in order* to "make it right". This was all to fix what I had done "wrong", from questioning.

Another desperate act to fix what I had done "wrong" was to delete the entire book I was writing from my laptop computer. I had been bashing religion and God. If the book "got out", it would have changed the world (so I thought). I had to apologize for what I had done. I even e-mailed a few people to tell them that God was punishing me, and I hoped he would have mercy on my soul.

It was the second night while watching the TV the sit-com "Friends", that the white people were turning black/dark. An overwhelming sensation of dread came over me. It was then that I decided to go to the hospital because I was going to die. I slowly made my way into the next room where my parents were watching TV. I told them I didn't feel good. They were watching 'Friends' also, and the characters where turning black/dark on their TV too. Slowly things all around me were turning dark. It seemed as if my perception was slowly fading away. I made another desperate attempt to go upstairs and beg God for forgiveness in private. I came back down stairs and hugged my Mother goodbye. I started crying and was saying that I was going to die. My step-dad drove, while my little brother was in the back seat. While we were driving, [to me] the radio in the car was turning on and off by itself, playing no specific songs—just music. Then "something said" I was going to die like my Father. At the last minute, as we were pulling in to the emergency area of the hospital, "something said" to save myself I had to ask my step-dad why he had made my sister feel uncomfortable growing up. When I did, "relief came over me". I jumped out of the car and crawled to the rear of the car, was on my knees screaming, at the top of my lungs, up to the star filled sky—full of joy. After I calmed down I noticed that my other brother and sister were there, standing outside. How did they get there (I asked myself)?

There were police there on duty. Everyone was trying to talk to me to get me to go into the emergency room. But now I had a "second chance at life". So now I was supposed to get back to my Mom and 'save' her and myself. I refused to go in. I had to get back home. My step-dad came over and confronted me. We then started to scuffle a little. "Something said" to **hit** him. But I couldn't do it. I guess I was able to still maintain just that *little bit* of control. Soon the police came over and started in with trying to maintain control of the situation. They were calmly talking to me to tell me to go in, since I was driven there for that reason in the first place. I decided to talk to my sister in private around the corner of the building. I told her that we needed to pray to Jesus together(I don't remember the rest). We walked back over to everyone else. Now I was really being pressured to go into the emergency room by everyone. I still refused. It was no good though, everyone surrounded me and the police grabbed me and handcuffed me. I started screaming again, but was talked into calming down. I was taken into an office and asked some questions (I don't remember). I think it was at this point that I viewed the police as "devils of this world". So I convinced them to take the handcuffs off, that I would cooperate. I was to see a Doctor first before they would let me leave. I was taken in the back and had to take my clothes off and put the gown on. My sister came in after. She was trying to talk to me. But my focus was on getting out of there. I had to get back to my Mother. As the policeman walked by the curtain, I stared at his eyes, noticing the blackness of his pupils. I was waiting for him to look away. When I got my chance, I lifted the curtain and ran for the door. My sister screamed at me to stop. I slammed through the door and practically knocked over a little old lady. The entrance was blocked with the police, my step-dad and my brothers. They immediately rushed me and tackled me to the floor. I was screaming that I was going to die and that I needed to see my Mother. My brother got in my face and was telling me to quit playing around (something like that). They got me up and took me in the back again. This time I was shackled at my wrists and ankles to the bed. A nurse came in and gave me two shots, one in each leg. She said it was going to help me calm down. Then a lady with a clipboard came in and started listening to me. I told her my thoughts were becoming frantic at this time. I had to see my Mom to tell her that I had to 'save' her and me, because I was going to die. I was then left alone. My mind was becoming desperate with solutions on how to get out of there. There was a little bit of blood coming out from where the shot was given in my right thigh. I stared at it and realized I had to start fighting to stay awake because I was going to die and wake up in hell. Then I just laid my head back and stared at the over-head light, quietly begging to Jesus and God for forgiveness and to save me.

THE HOSPITAL

I woke in the morning not knowing what the hell was going on. A voice came over the speaker system telling everyone that it was time to get up for breakfast. I was only wearing underwear and the garment from the night before. When I went down to the room where breakfast was being served, I grabbed a tray of food and noticed everyone was getting what they wanted. Mine was different for some reason; again, I had done something wrong.{Later, when the *reasoning* slowly came back into play, I eventually realized that at the end of each meal, we had menus to select the individual items we wanted for the same meal, just the next day.}

When I saw my Mother for the first time, I still had to do "that thing" for her and I. So I started to huff and puff and blow on my thumb so I could pass out. But as I was attempting to do this she called for the nurse and at the same time, "something said" not to scare her. She quickly departed the room, so I then stopped.

My first recollection of my surroundings was that I was stuck inside of a cross. The one long hallway intersected by the shorter one. And that there was no way out, except the locked and monitored glass door.

I was feeling physically very strange. I felt compelled to walk around, I didn't feel comfortable sitting down. When I did sit down, I just sat on the edge of the windowsill and looked out the window. I would think of why I was there. I didn't understand.

On the 3rd or 4th day when I saw my Mother again, I called her Mommy. She said, "I'm not your Mommy, I'm your Mother." I told her and my step-dad that I was feeling better. She commented back—it is because of the medication.

Another visit she brought me a crossword puzzle book to give me something to do. I wasn't able to figure it out though.

There was a schedule of activities each day listed on the board. Every hour or so there was something to do. We would do silly exercising while sitting in our chairs. Then other times we would do arts and crafts. {It was all to stimulate our minds, for our betterments.} We would all sit around in a circle and talk briefly about how each of us was doing that day. During relax times, I would just sit in the TV room and watch TV. I always felt physically disturbed, like I couldn't just sit still comfortably. I remember very well of the monitors that checked on each person about every 15 minutes or so.

I would talk to the Doctor briefly each day. He asked me how my thoughts were. I told him that things were slowly getting better (from what I can remember during that time). Every morning after breakfast I was given medications. Every night before bed, the same. Every other night or two I was awoken to someone taking blood from my arm. [It was to monitor the Depakote levels]. I do remember waking up one morning with the repeating question—why did Cain kill his brother Abel?

There was another visit by my Mother. She just stood around and didn't know what to say to me. Suddenly my neck became very stiff and it felt like my head wanted to twist off. I got scared and just sat down to figure out what was happening to me. The next thing I knew my Mother was gone. Later that night, when I went to lie down, my tongue started to twist on its own. I never experienced something like that before. I got up and told the nurse what was happening to me. He took me in a back room and gave me two shots in the ass. Whatever it was, it worked. I was able to get comfortable and sleep.

It must have been the 4th or 5th day there when I was told by the Doctor to call my Mom to have her come see me for my evaluation. When that day came, it was the Doctor, my Mom, my sister, a social worker, and myself in a room. He said that I had Bi-polar Schizophrenia. I had never heard of those words before. The diagnosis was a shock to me. I was a patient as involuntary status. If I wanted continued treatment, I had to stay and change to voluntary status. If I disagreed, I had no choice but to be involuntary status. No matter what, I wasn't going anywhere for a while.

I was given permission to go outside for a half an hour at a time, as long as I was escorted with another patient. When I got outside, I immediately looked for a way out. And I found one. There was just a chest-high wooden fence with an unlocked door to the parking lot and street. But for some funny reason, I "reasoned" that I shouldn't. I decided to play by the rules to get treated, and wait until I got discharged properly.

When the weekend came around I was given permission to leave the hospital under supervision for 6 hours on Saturday and 8 hours on Sunday. My sister came and got me. We went out to eat and bowling one of the days. Damn, I don't remember the other day. It doesn't matter. I was ok. I wanted to drink, out of habit, but of course wasn't supposed to and didn't.

After my weekend supervised, short retreats, I kept asking the Doctor when I was going to be able to be discharged. He said soon. I was obviously doing rather well.

AFTER DISCHARGE, GOING BACK TO FLORIDA

These are the times of not being able to concentrate worth a damn, because I was now a medicated zombie. I was instructed to take 2mg. of Risperdal, 500 mg. of Depakote, and 1mg. of Cogentine, for the side affects. I was to take these medications twice a day, until later evaluated by a new Doctor back in Florida.

The morning of my discharge *there was no one there for me.* I was given a bunch of medication and written directions to the mental health facility in St.Augustine, FL. My sister and other brother lived within walking distance from the hospital. So I walked over to their house and woke my brother up about 9am. My truck was parked in their driveway with all my stuff in it. It should have been at my parents house. I didn't know what to think. I felt no support from my parents. I stopped by my parents house the next day for dinner and then headed back to Florida the following day. I stopped off at my brother's apartment in VA Beach as a rest stop.

When I got back to Florida I was extremely afraid to be alone. I spent nearly a month falling asleep on my girlfriend's couch at her house. It was a very difficult time for both of us. I was very sensitive to noise. Everything seemed louder. If you have watched the movie 'A Beautiful Mind', it was very similar to what my girlfriend and I went through. I was the same way he was in the movie—heavily medicated and not able to respond and function properly. When we went to see that movie together, it brought back some unpleasant memories.

The medication was bringing me down terribly. All I wanted to do was sleep. I was sleeping a minimum of 12 hours a day. I was never completely focused. I don't remember exactly when, but I decided to only take my medication at bedtime. Because it was that bad to feel so sedated.

I remember waking up in the middle of the nights always afraid. It was like "something" was in the room with us. I would bury my head between the pillows and lie completely still. Then it sounded like 'that something' was scratching on the outside of the pillow. I would wake her up from time to time for comfort.

When I finally seen my first psychiatrist (since the hospital), I told him mostly about having read self-help books. It wasn't till the end of the session that I mentioned to him about being punished by God for having questioned the Bible. He said, "if that were true, half of society would be punished." That has stuck with me since. He also asked what religious background I was raised by. I told him Christian/Baptist. After consoling with my girlfriend about my session with the Doctor, she helped me understand why he asked me about my childhood religious upbringing.

After having been back in Florida for about 2 months, being unemployed and struggling mentally, I decided to pack up my belongings and move back to NY and live with my parents. It was just going to be temporary situation until I figured things out. For about a month, living in NY, I don't remember doing too much. I just hung out with my siblings and did a lot of sleeping.

FIRST RELAPSE, RECOVERY, BUT STILL STRUGGLING

I was back home living with my parents. It had only been about 3 months since my discharge from the hospital and being new to medication on a daily basis.

I was running low on medication and wondered if I needed it anymore. I made an appointment with a family medical Doctor to get a prescription for more medication. He asked me how I felt. I told him fine. He gave me a new prescription and, yet, told me I could wean off my medication. *He wasn't a psychiatrist.* And I didn't know any better.

It had been over a week since I had weaned down to 1mg. of Risperdal and had stopped taking the Depakote already. It was just a few days after stopping the 1mg. of Risperdal that it started to happen (now that I look back on it).

My little brother and I were upstairs in his room. He was playing on his computer, while we talked. I suddenly got a beautiful feeling of "goodness". When I was to go to bed, I was going to "converse" with God.

It was early July, and I became obsessed with having to visit my Father's grave for the first time in 23 years. I got my sister and her boyfriend to go with me to our relative's restaurant to get the directions to the grave. As I sat there talking with my Uncle, I was holding back some serious tears. He was on the phone with my Aunt and telling her that I was there visiting. I told him to tell her that I was sorry about the past (for a reason I don't remember). When we left the restaurant to go to the cemetery, I kept asking my sister if she really wanted to do the visit. I was supposed to do it by myself. That was the feeling persisting over me. When we finally found the grave, there was an "emotional block". I hadn't done it right, something was wrong.

Later that night, I was lying around with an uneasy stomach feeling. I had been slowly returning to watching church channels. Religion was over occupying my mind again. When I went to bed, I felt very uncomfortable. I wasn't able to rest comfortably. I saw an alien face; the typical large gray head with big black eyes, suddenly appear and then disappear. I was a little scared, but when it disappeared, I gave it no more thought. I tossed and turned with non-stop thoughts about how I had "not done it right" visiting the grave that day. I turned over and looked up at the window sill/curtains and saw some disfigured faces looking at me. I was disturbed and turned away. The next thing I noticed was a swirly pattern of lights around and above my head. My thoughts were telling me that I had only gotten it half right visiting the grave. I was apologizing for not having done it right. I eventually dozed off for maybe a couple of hours and woke up not feeling right (uneasy stomach). I ignored my irritability and pressed on with my plans of driving to VA Beach to stay with my brother. I was going to take time to try and figure out what I was going to do with my life next. My mind was thinking excessively again. As I drove down the highway, it was an analytical conversation going on in my head. I suddenly realized that I missed my exit. So I had to turn around and back track. I drove all the way to VA Beach with this state of mind. *It was an unpleasant drive.*

When I got to my brother's apartment I was non-stop thinking. I had thoughts of the story of Adam and Eve (again). Analyzing and obsessing, that's the only way to describe it. A thought "chimed in" saying, 'I didn't do it'[eat the forbidden fruit]. Then I got the inspiration that I could reverse what I had done to myself in Florida, in front of the mirror. So I went into the bathroom, in front of the mirror, and started talking to myself and crying again. I got frustrated and stopped. A conversation started, in my mind, about the makings of the Universe. And it wouldn't stop talking. I wasn't supposed to be thinking and knowing these thoughts, so I went outside to try and think of something else and talked to a neighbor. But it didn't help much. At a later time, I talked to another neighbor. I felt irritable. I was compelled to talk about God again. I would then feel elated. We went to his apartment and he got out the Bible and discussed it briefly. When I looked at the words on the page, they were "blocked/fuzzy" (that's the only way to describe it). As I was leaving, I remember a thought of getting to see God's face on the sun if I got up for the sunrise the next morning. After talking to the neighbor, I went back to the apartment, sat on the stairs, and just started crying for no particular reason.

While I was in VA Beach I was constantly questioning everyone I came across for their opinions/views on God. I would start to take walks up and down the boardwalk on the beach. When I was walking to the beach, one afternoon, I walked by a family standing near a bench. As I approached, the child dropped his ice cream cone. [To me] it was my fault (my bad presence). As I continued walking, I looked over to see large puppets that had strings attached to all their body parts to crossed-sticks above them—marionettes. I was attached "mentally the same way to God" as I looked at them.

One evening my brother and I were sitting outside having some food and talking. What was wrong with me at that time was, while I was trying to have a normal conversation with my brother—*my head was feeling estranged from my perception of the moment.* I was having constant unpleasant physical sensations in my head.

The idea of going to church again and talking to a preacher/priest came back at play with me. So I got up one morning and got dressed up and went to the nearest church. I remember analyzing the colors of the vehicles as I drove through the parking lot looking for a parking spot. I had a black truck, so black represented evil/bad. But I wasn't the only one with a black vehicle, but the point is *I analyzed and dwelled on it.* Services had just gotten out, so there were just a few people in the church. I asked a few people if there was a preacher I could talk to. I then realized there was one behind me. So I then asked him if I could speak to him in private. He sat me down and I then asked him, "does God punish people for questioning the Bible?" He looked at me a little funny and said, "no". He then asked me if I was hearing voices. I didn't know what he meant (at the time). I felt a little reassured and then left.

An afternoon at the Tavern having lunch with my brother, I was being bothered by a fly. I had to give it an "offering" to get it to leave me alone.

One evening on the way back from the Tavern, I was very uncomfortable with my persona. As my brother and I were walking down the road, I was thinking very deeply and I got a physical signal (from God) in my brain—and it was euphoric. I started to cry and actually stopped walking(and almost dropped to my knees). My brother had to pull me along, because he was afraid I was making a scene. I kept telling him how good I was feeling, as we walked back to the apartment.

Then there was an evening that my head was feeling physically strange. My brain had an uncomfortable physical sensation that wouldn't go away (that's the only way to describe it). I started praying to God for it to go away. But it didn't help. I sat there on the edge of the couch, like the cover of this book. I then tried to fall asleep feeling this way. I dozed off for just a short time, but was suddenly woken up to the sound of a slamming door. My head was feeling this strange sensation and *I thought and felt that I was in the presence of God.* I had prayed to God for my head sensations to go away, but the sound of the slamming door was God signaling no. My thoughts were taking over. I was "getting the message(s)"—I had to sign onto the Internet and start reading from the Bible again. I was supposed to read anything about Jesus. After a short time of reading, with my thoughts deciphering in a threatening way what I was reading, I went to sleep. But I woke up feeling bad.

The next night I lied down to go to sleep, but there was a conversation going on inside my head. I was talking to "another me". It wouldn't shut up. It just kept on talking back. I tossed and turned all night. The next thing I knew the sun was coming up. I was up before my brother was. He had to get ready and go to work. I told him I couldn't sleep. He was surprised, of course, that I was up and bothered by my problem. The first thing he said was, "take your medication, Dave". I ignored him and grabbed the phone book and started looking up mental health offices to go check into. {Its ironic that I knew something was wrong, but I wouldn't take my medication.} I drove to the psychiatric hospital in VA Beach at 630am and walked in to tell them I wasn't feeling good. She asked me a few questions and then sent me to the mental health department for evaluation. I was immediately questioned by a counselor and told to come back later for a talk with the psychiatrist. There was an opening that early afternoon, from a cancellation.

I don't even remember the conversation I had with the Doctor{sorry}. I told him that I had been on Risperdal and Depakote, and had stopped taking them. He gave me a new refill on both, and told me to follow up with the counselor in a couple days or so.

That night I took the medication and slept. The difference was obvious, looking back on it.

I began to be part of the VA Beach mental health system. Seeing the Doctor once a month and going to support meetings once a week. I was living with my brother and unemployed the whole time, but looking for work. It was a rough few months. I drove back and forth from VA Beach to Florida a couple times, during this time frame too. I wasn't able to figure things out on what to do with my life. I was still seeing my girlfriend at the time. We had been together at that point for over 3 years. She was there for me the best she could. I commend her for that.

During one of my visits with her she informed me of a movie that she watched a few days before my coming to visit her. She then insisted that I watch it with her. The movie is "Inherit the Wind". We watched the 1999 version. Her emphasis of me watching it was to see them questioning of the Bible in the courtroom at the end. I remember her telling me—see, they are questioning the Bible and they aren't being punished (by God). But the entire movie is excellent and shows the heavy debate between Religion and Evolution. It emphasizes the extreme fanaticism of religion against science.

When I was back in VA Beach I was struggling with sleeping too much and having obsessive thinking about Religion. I would talk to the fellow patients in the support group and ask them if they believed God would punish someone for questioning the Bible. I never got a straight answer. The point is, I obsessed about it still. I remember I was still so emotionally and physically distraught that, after the support group, I stopped by the church on the way home. I was alone in a private praying room and prayed to God for relief. I even left an offering in the plate.

I would take walks up and down the beach and start collecting trash and throw it away, thinking that I was collecting "brownie points" to get to heaven. A song that stuck with me at the time about how I thought God was thinking about me (in a negative way) was, "How you remind me" by Nickelback. When I saw the Doctor another time, he could tell I was in a depression and thinking too much. That's when I decided to start taking Zoloft. Within a week after starting the medication, of 50mg., I was feeling better.

Within a week I decided to go back to Florida and stay with my girlfriend again.

But shortly after I got back to Florida, I decided to leave again and go stay with my brother for a while. My girlfriend and I were just not working out anymore, so it was best to separate for a while. While I was in VA Beach I was looking for work again. An opening happened back at an old job in Melbourne, FL. I went there and worked for less than 2 weeks. Another old job back in St. Augustine, FL was supposedly opening back up, so I left Melbourne prematurely, before being confirmed of the new job. I ended up going back to VA Beach with my brother (again). I was jumping all over the place. It was unhealthy mentally and physically for me to be doing all that moving around.

Eventually I landed another aviation job at a company that I had worked before in the mid 90s. While I was there I had a hard time concentrating on my work. There was non-stop thinking happening all the time. I was experiencing deep, over-analytical thinking. The symptoms were still happening, barely tolerable, but I honestly couldn't take it anymore.

I was on the Internet one evening, reading about Bi-polar disorder, and suddenly became inundated with "confusion". I became very uncomfortable as my thoughts took over. Everything being said on the TV show that I was watching were "special messages" to me from God. I just lied there and didn't know what to do. A thought dominated me by suggesting that God was giving me a second chance, if I were to read the Bible again. I eventually fell asleep, but was woken up in the middle of the night feeling uneasy. I went into work the next day, but had a hard time concentrating. I remember reading something and feeling as if it were a subliminal message from God. Then while I was attempting to work, my thoughts became so deep and analytical that I wasn't able to concentrate on my job. I decided to leave and go back to the hotel room and take my medication. As I was walking through the parking lot, I was completely uneasy. I was having a very hard time, to put it bluntly. I was so disturbed at that point that when I got back to my hotel room, I called my girlfriend to tell her how I was feeling.

It was just a couple of weeks until Christmas. I wanted to go home as I had always done in the past. I quit the job and told the boss I would be back after the holidays. I was a con-tract/temporary employee so he agreed that I could come back if I wanted to. When I started driving back to VA Beach, I drove past the exit, 58 east to VA Beach, by about 20 miles. My mind was so pre-occupied that I wasn't able to pay attention.{That's a moderate symptom}.

My brother and I drove back together to NY for Christ-mas. What I can remember most from the drive was being too quiet for my brother. He wanted conversation to help pass the time and make the drive more pleasant. I had a lit-tle trouble listening to music. I was too focused on listening to the words, that I wasn't truly enjoying the essence of the music.

When we got to our parents house I had gone above the garage to go through some things of mine that I had stored there. I noticed my stuff had been moved and wondered why. When my step dad came by to say HI, he told me an incident that had happened with my stuff, to explain why it had been moved. He said that it had rained really hard one day and that the roof leaked exactly where my stuff was. Immediately I interpreted it as another "bad doing (by God)" intentionally to me, and I got moderately unnerved.

It was the holiday season so I decided to have a few beers. I also decided to skip taking my medications at bedtime after an evening of drinking. I seemed to be fine, until the third morning. When I woke up in the morning with light being in the room, I saw small "things" floating and slowly rotating around in the air. It's very hard to describe what I saw. But one description is to compare it to a chandelier. From time to time the "things" would change. I closed my eyes and turned over to hope that they would go away. But even with my eyes closed, I could see them. The next "thing" I saw was a small face of some kind looking at me, slowly moving around the edge of the pillows of the couch. Then something was said to me in thought—we are waiting for you. Now I was getting an uneasy sensation that something wasn't quite right (obviously). So I got up and took my medication and fell back to sleep. I felt better later that morning.

Later that day I told my Mother that I had hallucinated that morning because I had purposely skipped my medication. Her and my step-dad asked what I had seen. I tried to describe it. But they emphasized that I was wrong for doing that to myself, by not taking my medications. When our visit ended and I hugged my Mother good-bye, I simply remember her telling me—don't stop taking your medications.

BACK TO WORK AND WEANING OFF THE MEDICATIONS, UNSUCCESSFULLY

I had been living with my brother for a few months in VA Beach. I had seen the Doctor once a month, gone to support groups once a week, and taken my medications on a daily basis. Unfortunately, the only thing I did was sleep. I would sleep for over 12 hours a day, sometimes all day. There were days I never even left the apartment. I still struggled mildly from symptoms, but I was able to function. It was during this time frame that I had weaned down to 1mg. of Risperdal and 250mg. of Depakote.

I had been looking for work in VA Beach still. But one day I was on the Internet and noticed a job had opened up back at a prior employer in St.Augustine, FL. I applied for it and gotten accepted to go back. What a relief, to get a job after being out of work for nearly a year (minus the few weeks in Florida and North Carolina). When I had gotten back to work at the prior job in St.Augustine, FL, in the beginning of 2002, I checked into the mental health department for medication management. I saw the Doctor once a month. There were no support groups that I was informed of at the time.

When I got back to working on a daily basis, I wasn't in my usual morning routine. I usually would shower in the mornings before work. Instead, I showered at night before bed. I would get up and hardly brush my hair and go into work. My point of mentioning this is, that I was not my usual self. We all do our usual routines. I wasn't able to do what I usually did.

Then there were times I would test my medications. I would skip taking it a couple days in a row. I remember one night I had a very detailed dream about my brother yelling at me and telling me what was real and what wasn't. I was woken up to feeling very confused and scared. I got up and saw a shadow in the window that resembled a dinosaur head with big sharp teeth. And when I saw it I got the shivery sensations in my head (again). I took my medications and went back to sleep.

When I started going to the local Library, I would have trouble picking out certain books that I wanted to read. I would be nervous to pick up religious related books. I remember having trouble reading a little. Thoughts would intrude at times.

One time while I was just lying on the couch relaxing, hallucinating came back to play with me. As I was looking at the wall, I watched the patterns change form and move around the wall on their own. It was a very strange experience for me.

I remember a day that I was running errands. On my way back to my apartment I actually drove around in circles, because I couldn't make up my mind due to my "continuous" (racing) thoughts.

Another lay off came. But I and another guy were spared. And then we changed departments. That was a good thing, to still be employed. It was shortly after I changed jobs there that I decided to wean off my medication, under supervision of my psychiatrist. For some strange reason I wanted to see if I truly had this "problem". I was down to 1mg. of Risperdal, and 250mg. of Depakote, and 50mg. of Zoloft. I was to wean of the Zoloft first, according to the Doctor. After just a couple weeks of weaning down to 25mg and then stopping, I noticed the differences. I had a hard time getting up in the mornings for work. I became a very grumpy person. And drinking too much came back into play. (I substituted the alcohol with the absence of the Zoloft, without realizing it). I thought I could adjust to the irritability and continue on with the weaning off with the next medication, Risperdal. How wrong I was.

During this time frame I was on .5mg of Risperdal, *every other day*, with the 250mg. of Depakote.

Ruminating thinking started back up. I was constantly over-analyzing the creation story of Adam and Eve in Genesis from the Bible. I began to think about God too much and whether he existed or not. And I had a hard time reading. I would get a lot of headaches too.

There was a day at work when I was conversing with a fellow employee and "something" was intruding in my thoughts, telling me that he was holding back his laughter from our talking. This forced me to have a hard time making eye contact, because I was also holding back from just bursting out laughing.

One of the other employees would always wear this T-shirt that had two dragons facing each other, on the back. I would always construe it as the battle between good and evil.

During the weekend my girlfriend wanted me to watch a video with her. It was the movie "A.I.". I remember being uncomfortable watching it. I actually had to turn away from the screen sometimes. My mind was analyzing everything in a religious framework. I also remember feeling physically slightly detached from reality; it was eerie.

There was an afternoon that my girlfriend and I went to the local Library to relax and read a bit; that I had an obvious episode that she witnessed. I had picked up a book and started reading about schizophrenia. While I was reading a sentence, a "thought replaced/inserted" what I was reading, and then I got a physical sensation in my brain. I became so disturbed by this that I had to stop reading and put the book down. She saw something was wrong. But it still didn't click for me to realize I was having symptoms again.

When I would be over at my girlfriend's sister's home, I was back to constantly bringing up topics of God and the Bible. I was drinking a lot again to try and make myself feel better when we were all together. Then when we went to bed that evening, I was having strange, uncomfortable sensations in my head. I guess at that point I realized I was relapsing and needed my medication. It was about 4am. I got up, dressed and drove back to my apartment, in a "very strange" and paranoid frame of mind. I took my medications and went to bed. Later that morning, I met my friends at the beach, but I felt "different". I was better, but "different". The only way to describe "different" is to say that I felt helpless and not being able to feel confident and comfortable.

When I saw the Doctor again just a few days later, he noticed I was struggling. He asked me why I was doing this to myself. He made me realize that I needed my medications and that it wasn't my fault that I had this problem.

So I went back on my medications to the prior dosages: .5mg. Risperdal, 250mg. Depakote, and 50mg.

Zoloft—daily. The differences came immediately. The first time I noticed feeling better was an afternoon with my girlfriend, at her sister's home. We were all together and I suddenly realized I was not obsessing about God, the Bible, and anything religious. She told me that it had already been mentioned that they noticed the differences in me, and that I was doing better. Getting back on the Zoloft at 50mg. initially gave me some side affects. So I went down to 25mg. and I felt better. The Zoloft works for me on the obsessive thinking and the depression at the same time. What a wonderful medication it is. Risperdal is the anti-psychotic medication that keeps me from being delusional and not hallucinating. Depakote is the mood stabilizer that keeps me from becoming hyper-manic, which would start with elation and then escalate. A note here—the medications do not cure the condition/illness, they just treat the symptoms.

A NEW JOB

An opportunity presented itself for me to go to a new job. I was a temporary/contract employee with no benefits with the same aerospace corporation for over three years (on and off) and going nowhere. I needed health insurance. That was the first thing on my mind. I wanted therapy. I needed to be able to talk to a psychologist about my experiences.

After a couple months from my application, the paper work for my security clearance came back good. I was a little worried about getting approved because of my recent past, having been in the psych ward for psychiatric problems. I got a start date of Sept. 27, 2002. I gave a week's notice to the boss. I emphasized how much I wanted to stay and be a permanent employee with benefits and live in Florida. But he said they could do nothing for me about that. So I realized I had a better opportunity with the new employer.

I have started new jobs several times before, so it wasn't too difficult to adjust. None of my fellow employees at the new employer knows of my mental condition (but now they will). I checked into the community mental health clinic for medication management, because my health insurance wasn't available till after the 90-day probation period from the company.

Looking back at the probation period and until I saw my new therapist and new psychiatrist, I was still having very mild symptoms and was only lightly aware of them. Things people said had a "special and different kind" of meaning for me. I was back to testing my medications on a weekend basis. Again and again I would go to bed after a night of drinking on the weekends without taking my medications. And again and again I would wake up in the middle of the night feeling bad. My brother and close friend would give me shit on the phone on why I was doing that to myself. The people who where getting to know me at work said I was a very pessimist person. I got a reputation real fast as being Mr. Doom and Gloom. I was rather moody and complained a lot about things out of my control. A few people from time to time asked me if I was Bi-polar. I had to bite my tongue and not comment. I didn't want to people to know that I was actually more complicated than just being Bi-polar(having the Schizophrenia mix too, equaling Schizo-affective).

CHRISTMAS 2002, PARANOIA

When I had gone back home to visit my family for the Christmas holiday, I was drinking moderately and testing my medication a couple of nights in a row by not taking it at bedtime (like I'm supposed to). One night I was abruptly woken up to my brother talking to me. But he wasn't, he was still sleeping.

As a present to my sister and her boyfriend for Christmas, my brother and I agreed to play some tricks on them. They are both smokers. And cigarette prices had jumped up very high in the state of NY. So as we passed through the state of Pennsylvania we bought a carton of cigarettes for quite a bit cheaper than if bought in NY. So the trickery was going to done the whole time I was there. When we were all out drinking and having fun, and my sister and her boyfriend weren't looking, I would replace a brand new pack of cigarettes with theirs, when it was just about empty. I did a few other simple tricks to make them question things. It was fun doing this. And it worked. But I was getting this "feeling" at the same time that I wasn't supposed to be doing this kind of stuff during Christmas. On Christmas Eve I went to bed after a night of partying and moderate drinking and *not* taking my medication. I woke up feeling "not right". My brother and I shared the same room while staying at my sister and boyfriend's apartment. He wasn't in his bed. Where was he? I was alone. My thoughts were starting to take over and paranoia setting in. I wasn't supposed to be playing those cigarette tricks during Christmas. Playing tricks was supposed to be only done on Halloween. I started to apologize. I started to hear a lot of cracking noises throughout the apartment. My perception was shifting to fear again. I got up and went into the next room to see if my brother was Ok. He had drank too much from the night before and went to lie down in the other room. I went into the bathroom to try and figure out what was happening. But the "noises that go bump in the night" were coming to get me. I heard the door in the next room open. But right when I was beginning to over react, the cat came strolling in. I was stuck in between **extreme paranoia** and rationalizing things out. It was time to take my medication and lie back down to try and sleep. I took my medication and, I literally felt the "uneasy physical sensations and paranoia" start going away. My perception started to shift back to normal and I went back to sleep. In the morning when I told my brother what I experienced the night before, he said I was wrong for not taking my medication. He talked to his friend on the phone on what I had told him about what I went through and said, "its not bad or/and wrong to be playing cigarette tricks during Christmas." {What do you the reader think?}

NEW DOCTORS

When I saw my first psychologist and psychiatrist on bene-fits from my new employer, they each came to the immedi-ate conclusions that I wasn't on the proper dosage of medication. The maintenance dosage of Risperdal for Schizo-affective is 1mg. I had been on .5 mg. for several months. I had weaned down that low and just assumed that that's all I needed when going back on it. Again, I was wrong and the Doctors' right. But I was stubborn and decided to go see another psychiatrist for a second opinion. Going up on medication was something that I didn't want to hear. When I saw the new Doctor, I told him of my med-ication and other Doctor's advice. He then asked me how many Doctors I was going to go see until I heard what I wanted to hear (which wasn't going to happen, anyhow). I got frustrated with him too and left. I went back to the first psychiatrist and decided to do my part, which he liked to call being "medication compliant".

It was because of the few things I told the Doctors about incidents that I had in my apartment, that they didn't like, that forced me to realize that I was still borderline delusional at times.

I was on the phone with my girlfriend an afternoon after seeing my special friend the two nights in a row, prior. I was hung over still too. When she described the details of where I had been with the other woman, the power went out and the phone connection was lost (cordless phone); but it came back on within a few seconds. To me, it was a bad signal from God. My thoughts started to take over and I got very nervous. I got so worried about it that I went to the neighbor and asked if he was having electrical problems too. He was. So I slowly got to thinking that I wasn't being singled out.

I was having computer modem problems (high speed Internet). When the cable guy came to trouble shoot the problem, I thought it was "my fault". He said the line in the living room was burnt and had a week signal. It was Ok for the TV cable, but not good for high-speed Internet use, as he put it. A lightning strike may have caused the problem. He mentioned several other possibilities. But I started to over analyze and dwell on the reason, and think back to that day the power went out temporarily. I thought it was a bad sign from God (for being bad).

Then there was a time at work when I was standing with my co-workers at the end of the shift, that I had an incident and one of them looked at me funny because of what I experienced. I was in the middle of a conversation and my thoughts got "temporarily deep" and then I got a vibrating sensation on my right hip. It startled me so, that I stopped and grabbed my side. It was the same exact vibrating I get from my cell phone when I have it on my hip. Except, I wasn't wearing it!!! Then my mood dropped and I felt uncomfortable for a few hours after that, worrying about it.

Sometimes when I would watch TV, I would get mild physical sensations in my brain. It would mostly happen during exciting, stimulating scenes. I remember very well it happened when I was drinking at a restaurant with new friends, watching the SuperBowl.

When I had my next Doctor's visit, I finally agreed to go up to the proper dosage of the Risperdal to 1mg. There was an immediate difference, but not comfortable either. It was making me almost oversleep in the mornings of having to go to work. And then while at work I was feeling a little "disconnected". I didn't like it and was getting worried that I was going to be this way permanently. So I started to chip off .25mg of the pills. I was at .75mg. instead of 1mg. Within a few days I started to feel better. Looking back on it, I just never gave my mind a chance to adjust to the new, recommended dosage. I stayed on .75mg. Risperdal for over six months, even though my Doctor insisted that I take the whole (1mg.) pill instead of chipping it off that little bit. He called me extremely stubborn. But I noticed the positive difference without any doubt.

When the holidays approached I began to stress over my travel plans and family affairs for Christmas. A few nights in a row, in the last week of November, I had unusual sleep disturbances. And at work I had mood swings that were noticeable to my fellow employees. When I saw my Doctor the first week of December and told him of my mild problems, he finally convinced me to take the whole pill (1mg.) of Risperdal. I also told him that I had been stressing. He said that stress triggers the symptoms.

During my second night's sleep, on the new higher dosage of Risperdal, I had a bad episode. I had a bad, vivid dream about death and going to heaven and hell. I woke up with my heart pounding fast and hard. I had the feeling of "God influence/control over me". The feeling was in a negative way. My thoughts were "strong" and they raced. And I got the feeling of staying awake 'forcefully'. But the episode lasted briefly and it went away. I noticed it was just five minutes until the alarm was going to turn on. So I got up and started my morning routine getting ready for work with mild anxiety. When I went to work my mood was irritable and uncomfortable for most of the day. I was asked if I was Ok. I just replied that I had a bad morning. It bothered me enough to call my Doctor and have him call me when I got home. When we talked on the phone later that day he told me that it can happen without notice. But stress is what triggers it. Was it my stressful dream? *When it happened, I was no longer in "control".*

The holidays passed with a nice family visit back to NY. And I noticed even a more positive difference on the 1mg. of Risperdal.

EARLY WARNING SIGNS OF SCHIZOPHRENIA

People whose family members have schizophrenia developed the following list of warning signs. Many behaviors described are within the range of normal responses to situations. Yet families sense—even when symptoms are mild—that behavior is "unusual"; that the person is not the same.

The number and severity of these symptoms differ from person to person—although almost everyone mentions "noticeable social withdrawal". The *italicized* words are what happened to me.

- *Hearing and seeing things that aren't there*
- Deterioration of personal hygiene
- Depression
- Bizarre behavior
- *Irrational statements*

- Sleeping excessively or *inability to sleep*
- Social withdrawal, isolation, and reclusiveness
- *Shift in basic personality*
- Unexpected hostility
- Deterioration of social relationships
- *Hyperactivity* or inactivity—or alternating between the two
- *Inability to concentrate* or to cope with minor problems
- *Extreme pre-occupation with religion*
- Excessive writing without meaning
- *Indifference*
- Dropping out of activities—or out of life in general
- Forgetting things
- Extreme reactions to criticism
- *Inability to express joy*
- Inability to cry, or *excessive crying*
- Inappropriate laughter
- *Unusual sensitivity to stimuli (noise, light, colors, textures)*
- Drug or alcohol abuse

- Fainting
- Strange posturing
- Refusal to touch persons or objects; wearing gloves, etc.
- Cutting oneself; threats of self-mutilation
- Staring without blinking—or blinking incessantly
- Peculiar use of words or odd language structures
- Sensitivity and irritability when touched by others

DSM-IV Criteria

Bi-polar disorder has its own set of symptoms. It is characterized by an alternating pattern of emotional highs (mania) and lows (depression). But a few are similar to schizophrenia, in its severest cases.

In the Manic phase, the signs and symptoms include:

- Feelings of euphoria, extreme optimism and inflated self-esteem
- Rapid speech, racing thoughts, agitation and increased physical activity
- Poor judgement and recklessness
- Difficulty sleeping
- Tendency to be easily distracted
- Inability to concentrate
- Extreme irritability

In the Depression phase, the signs and symptoms include:

- Persistent feelings of sadness, anxiety, guilt or hopelessness
- Disturbances in sleep and appetite
- Fatigue and loss of interest in your daily activities
- Difficulty in concentrating
- Recurring thoughts of suicide

CONCLUSION

When I look back on it now from nearly 3 years ago, of the diagnosis, it all makes sense. It has taken this time for me to accept the facts, listen to the Doctors, and test my medications, to realize that I have a mental condition/illness. How do I deal with such a thing in my life? I deal with it by doing what I have to do. I take my medications on a daily basis. For me, daily dosages of Risperdal(1mg) and Depakote(250mg.) at bedtime, and Zoloft(37.5mg) in the morning, keep me sane and stable. I still drink very socially on the weekends. Even though I know I'm not supposed to, according to the Doctors. I don't believe in total abstinence of alcohol. I just have to be careful. I don't question my condition anymore. I have accepted it.

I have been told that some never come out of their psychosis. I can say that I can imagine that, because I have been there. And an unfortunate way out of that "hell" (without help/medication) is eventual suicide. Even I contemplated it.

Because of what I have experienced I definitely have a different view on life, especially religion. I could go on and on about the subject of religion, but that would be another book. A close friend, who I confided with about my (psychotic) experiences related to God and religion, commented back saying—people who speak (directly) with or/and receive (special) messages/visions from God, back then they [society] made them prophets; nowadays we medicate (and commit) them. With that being said, my imagination and intellect makes me ponder about human history and psychosis; because back then they didn't have medications like we have nowadays to treat the condition. Was the condition a problem and labeled "evil", or was it exceptional and labeled "divine inspiration" and worshiped? It must have just depended on which culture you lived in.

Pre and early written history of cultures and their beliefs makes me speculate where they got their inspirations. Remember, Joan of Arc was "hearing voices and having visions from God". She led the battles with reverence from the church. But then she was considered a heretic and burned at the stake. How ironic!!!

I remember my Mother telling me how fortunate I am for having medications that work for me. Again, I can only imagine how I would have been treated just five hundred years ago. Considering how *superstitious and ritualistic* societies were (and still are), at first I would have been extolled, but then I would have been exorcized or/and put to death.

Newsweek ran a cover story on March 11, 2002 about Schizophrenia. The following is excerpt from that story.

"Whether it brings the voices of heaven or hell, it causes what must surely be the worst affliction a sentient, conscious being can suffer: the inability to tell what is real from what is imaginary. To the person with schizophrenia the voices and visions sound and look as authentic as the announcer on the radio and the furniture in the room.

"The seeming authenticity of the voices means that people with schizophrenia can be barraged by commands that, they are convinced, come from God or Satan. That inference is not illogical: who else can speak to you, unseen, from inside your head? Some patients have heard commands to shoplift, some to commit suicide. Believing she was possessed by Satan, [Andrea] Yates thought that her children "were not righteous." If she killed them while they were young, she told a psychiatrist, then "God would take them" up to heaven. Legally, "insanity" means the inability to tell right from wrong. There is no evidence that people with schizophrenia have impaired moral judgement. Then why do some obey commands to break the law, or worse? Perhaps one need look no further than Genesis 22. When Abraham heard God's command to sacrifice his only son, Isaac, he did not hesitate to take the boy up the mountain to the place of sacrifice and raise the knife."

Makes you think, does it not?

OCCAM'S RAZOR

A rule in science and philosophy stating that entities should not be multiplied unnecessarily. This rule is interpreted to mean that the simplest of two or more competing theories is preferable and that an explanation for unknown phenomena should first be attempted in terms of what is already known. *And to simplify it even more, it means that the simplest explanation is usually the correct one.*

I use this statement to help me rationalize what happened to me. When I was in psychosis, I was no longer "myself". For reasons not yet understood, my brain's chemistry malfunctioned, causing thoughts that weren't mine and not valid (delusions). I *had* to do things that I would not do otherwise (loss of control). I perceived sights and sounds that weren't there (hallucinations). And my emotions (affect) were amplified to the point of inappropriateness.

Hyper-religiosity is a product of Schizophrenia. The overall theme of my psychosis was persecution from God, for having questioned the Bible. It had taken lots of talks with those close to me, as well as therapy, to know that that is **not** true. Therapy made me realize that I was not on the proper dosage of Risperdal. It was therapy that helped me realize that when I have thoughts (about anything), to think about them and not be afraid. And therapy helped me realize that when I have questions, to ask and not be afraid.

I was questioning Life and God. And I still do. *Life is about questioning anything and everything.* I use Occam's Razor to help explain the meaning of life (in my view).

AFTERWORDS

This condition is a biological-chemical imbalance in the brain. **I felt it, so I know.** It affects the thinking processes to the point where one loses control and touch with reality. *Perception changes.* Paranoia, fear, and guilt set in to make me feel like doing nothing. Noises become louder and take on new meanings, with a combination of not knowing if what I'm hearing is real or not. Obsessive, over-analytical thinking consumes my mind. Not being able to read (correctly) is a result. Anything being said, anywhere, becomes subliminal messages. Shadows and points of light are seen in the peripheral visions that distract me at first; then they come more into direct view. Visions come into view when I wake up from disturbed sleep when more time passes. Not being able to sleep is a symptom, which in turn complicates the problem. And the physical discomfort becomes excruciating; yet with exhilaration other times. Need I say more? That's what happens to *me*, if I stop taking my medications.

I know the differences between reality and delusions, because of my medications. And for being stable long enough. There are times that I get a little confused and uneasy, but its part of my life now.

I thank science and medicine for the help they are giving to the people who are experiencing this problem; so that most of us affected can live normal and healthier lives. For if it was not for science and medicine, my life would have ended as I knew it, and this book would not have been written.

When I started writing this book at the beginning of 2003, I was "uneasy" recalling what happened to me. Concluded at the beginning of 2004, it has actually been rather therapeutic. I no longer question taking my medications. I know that I have to take them (daily).

During the summer of 2003, the number one song then, that corresponds a little bit to what this book is about is from Matchbox 20, called "Unwell". The video shows him having hallucinations. Although it's just a glimpse of how horrible the symptoms truly are. My girlfriend, at the time, told me that it is a song from my perspective. I thought the same thing when I first heard it.

I started at my (new) present job in September of 2002. I am a permanent, full-time employee with the nation's number one aerospace defense contractor, as an electrical installer, building the newest stealth, fighter/attack jet for the U.S. Air force. I work out 3 days a week. And live alone in a one-bedroom apartment. I have my friends at work, so I socialize very well. I am considered to be a very successful person living with a mental condition (according to my

Doctors), as long as I take my medications. I will probably be on my medications for the rest of my life. I have been told (by the Doctors) that I should simply compare myself to a diabetic. A diabetic requires medication everyday too, for their condition.

The book Surviving Schizophrenia (4th edition) by E. Fuller Torrey, M.D. became my 'Bible' for a long time after my "breakdown". Everything that happened to me is correlated in that book. Page 40 is the best, detailed description of another person's experience that happened to me also. It's a *perfect* book for better understanding this problem.

I hope this book has helped others, similar to me, realize and understand that they are not alone. And I hope this book has erased a lot of the stigma and misunderstandings of mental illness for the rest of society.

Of all the reading I have done on the Internet concerning this subject in regards to religion, two web pages have stood out the most to me, thus far.

http://webpages.charter.net/blueskies24/_spiritchat/0000028a.htm

http://www.jcnot4me.com/Items/Misc%20Topics/schizophrenia_and_personal_revelations.htm

REFERENCES

DSM-IV

Surviving Schizophrenia (4th edition) by E. Fuller Tor-rey, M.D.

Newsweek, March 11, 2002

Contact me via E-mail: DavidCBoyles@Aol.com

0-595-30494-X

Printed in the United States
102350LV00001B/135/A

9 780595 304943